# Keto Diet

*Keto Diet and Ketogenic Kept Simple with 20 Simple Keto Recipes (Low-Carb, High-Fat), A Great Keto Cookbook For Weight-Control, Great Health And Well Being.*

The information herein is offered for informational purposes solely and is universal as so. The presentation of the information is without a contract or any type of guarantee assurance.

The trademarks that are used are without any consent, and the publication of the trademark is without permission or backing by the trademark owner. All trademarks and brands within this book are for clarifying purposes only and are the owned by the owners themselves, not affiliated with this document.

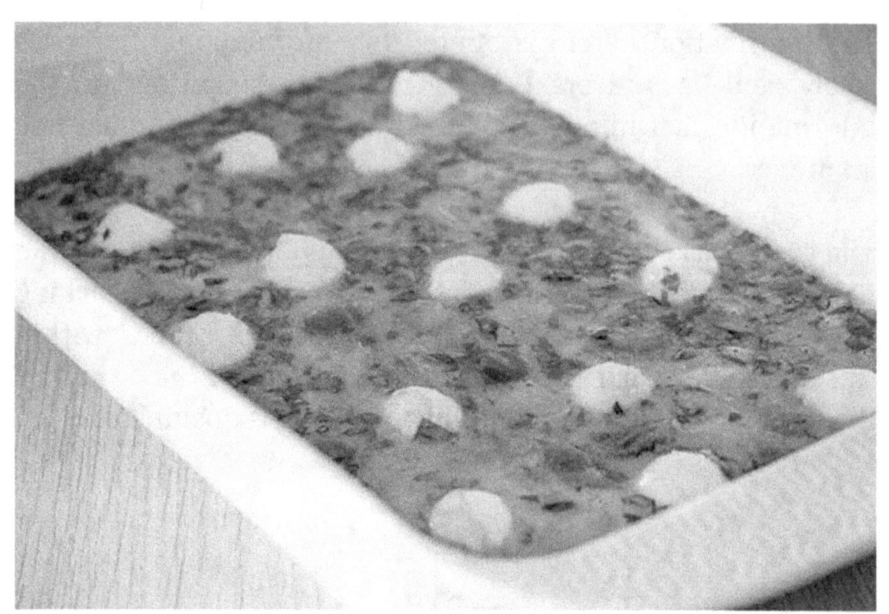

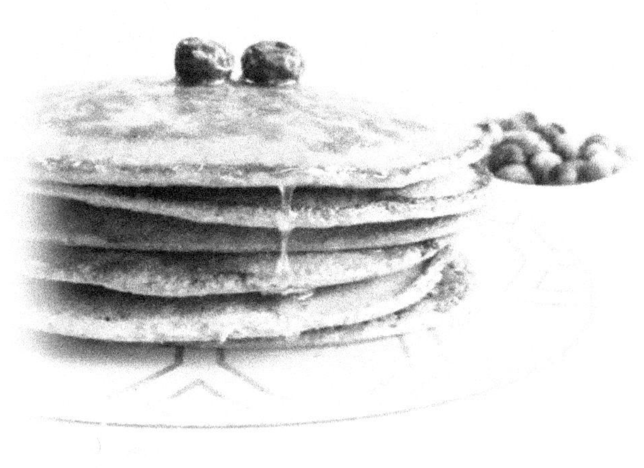

Other books by this Publisher *Awere First Publishing:-*

- GO TO our website: www.awerefirstpublishing.com OR check on ourlist OR https://amzn.to/2I6fpoe

- ALSO, you can follow us on our various *Social Media Platforms*:-

  o **PINTEREST**: kindlebooks8566

  o **YouTube**: AwereFirstPublishing CHANNEL

  o **LINKEDIN**: linkedin.com/in/awerefirst-publishing-26870417b

  o **TWITTER:** https://twitter.com/Awerefirstpubl1

  o (Audiobook_samples)**SOUNDCLOUD**: www.soundcloud.com/awerefirstpublishing


- This book is **NOW AVAILABLE** on AUDIOBOOK...**!!!**

  o Audiobook available**...on iTUNES (https://apple.co/2YT6DYH)**

  o Audiobook available**...on Audible.co.uk(UK), Audible.com(US), Audible.fr(FR), Audible.de(DE)**

  o Audiobook available**...on AMAZON**

**Table of Contents**

# Introduction

I want to thank you and congratulate you for downloading the book, *‘Keto Diet: Keto Diet and Ketogenic kept simple with 20 simple keto recipes (low-carb, high-fat), a great keto cookbook for weight-control, great health and well being.'*

Most people are driven by a need to do better in life in every way possible. They want to be wealthier and have more than the next person; however, doing well in life should also include being as healthy as possible. A lot of people take their health for granted until it is too late. If you are reading this, you probably want to pay more attention to your wellbeing now, and it is never too late.

One of the most common ailments that makes people conscious of their health is being overweight. It is easy to gain excess weight, as there are many junk and unhealthy food available around us, which we easily succumb to. If you want to lose that weight or want to pay more attention to your body, you need to keep some things in mind.

The first is to avoid any fad diets that people might rave about because these will usually harm you rather than do any good. A lot of such diets will ask you to eat less or eat only a few things. This prevents your body from getting the essential nutrients it requires. Instead, choose a healthier option like the ketogenic diet.

You might have heard of the ketogenic diet, but may not have all the information you need to know how it helps you. I will tell you exactly what it is and how it will benefit your health in the first chapter of the book.

I have also put together 20 amazing recipes to help you get started on this diet. Rest assured that you wouldn't have to starve yourself or count calories while on the ketogenic diet. Just follow the simple rules of the diet and add some exercise to your daily routine, eat sustainably and remain healthy to enjoy all the benefits of your hard work.

Thanks again for downloading this book, I hope you enjoy it!

# Chapter One: About the Ketogenic Diet

The ketogenic or keto diet as it is commonly known advocates the consumption of high amounts of fat and fewer carbohydrates. It might sound surprising, as we tend to believe that eating high amount of fat doesn't exactly sound healthy. But trust me when I say this, this diet is going to work for you if you follow it the right way.

Researchers have conducted a lot of studies on the keto diet, and most people have seen positive results. Unlike other diets, it won't be too hard to follow or restrict you from eating when you're hungry. Food is essential for the body's wellbeing and starvation is never the solution to get a fit body. You probably think that any fat is bad for you, but there are two types of fat, the good fat and bad fat. The solution is not to avoid all fatty food. The problem with the processed food that we eat is it contains unhealthy preservatives and components that are not good for your body.

Refined sugar is one of the main culprits that lead to obesity. The keto diet asks you to cut off refined sugar as much as possible since it has no nutritive value. This is easy when you stop buying too much-processed food from the stores and instead eat a more wholesome diet. Throw away all the sugar-laden cereals and candies from your pantry.

Instead, stock up on more healthy fruit, vegetables and meat that you can use to prepare your meals. This will allow you to be more conscious of what you are consuming. Over time, you will also notice a difference in how your body looks and feels. Refined sugar can make you lazy and tire you out after the initial sugar rush. Instead, the keto diet will help you feel energetic all day and get a good night's rest.

Your diet is essential for a healthy lifestyle. When you follow the keto diet, you will eat more fat and fewer carbohydrates. This will make your body go into a state of ketosis. Ketosis refers to the state your body goes through when it doesn't have access to carbs (glucose).

As you know, your body requires energy. During ketosis, glucose is not the primary energy source it usually is. Fats are turned into ketones in the liver, and the body uses these as a source of energy. This is how more fat is burned during when you follow this diet instead of it getting stored. Eventually, the stored fat in your body will also start converting into ketones and be utilized. This is how you will see a loss in excess weight in your body.

Since carbohydrates are only required in a certain amount by the body, reducing it will not cause any harm. Another benefit of the keto diet is that you won't suffer from hunger pangs and cravings. Too much carbohydrate consumption leads to feeling hungry more often. A healthy keto meal will leave you satisfied till your next appropriate mealtime. If you don't overeat, you will not gain excess weight. Thus, the keto diet helps to keep your weight under check.

To make your ketogenic journey easy, I have collated 20 interesting and healthy ketogenic recipes that will help you get started. So, without further ado, let's move to the recipes.

# Breakfast Tacos

Preparation time: 15 minutes

Cooking time: 15 minutes

Number of servings: 2

Nutritional values per serving:

Calories – 360, Fat – 29 g, Carbohydrate – 4 g, Net Carbohydrate – NA, Protein – 20 g

## Ingredients:

- 2 large eggs
- 4 slices pastured bacon, sugar free
- 6 ounces aged Cheddar cheese, shredded
- 2 teaspoons ghee
- 1 cup arugula
- Salt to taste
- Black pepper powder to taste
- ¼ teaspoon turmeric powder
- 4 sprigs fresh cilantro, chopped

## Method:

1. Place a nonstick pan over medium heat. Add bacon and cook until crisp. Remove bacon with a slotted spoon and set aside on a plate lined with paper towels.
2. Place a nonstick pan over medium heat. Add 1-teaspoon ghee. When the ghee melts, scatter half the cheese in a round shape.
3. Cook until the cheese melts. Crack an egg in the middle of the cheese circle.
4. Season with salt, pepper and turmeric powder.

5. When the egg is slightly cooked, cover with a lid that is tight fitting. Cook for about 2 minutes or until the egg is cooked and the cheese is crisp.
6. Carefully slide the taco on to a plate. Lift 2 opposite sides of the cheese round and hold it for a while so that it dries and acquires the shape of a taco. It can be done using 2 bowls. Place, one on each side, below the cheese so that the sides get lifted.
7. Fill one of the tacos with half the bacon and half the arugula.
8. Sprinkle half the cilantro and serve.
9. Repeat steps 2-8 to make the other taco.(**figure. 1**)

Figure 1.  Breakfast Tacos

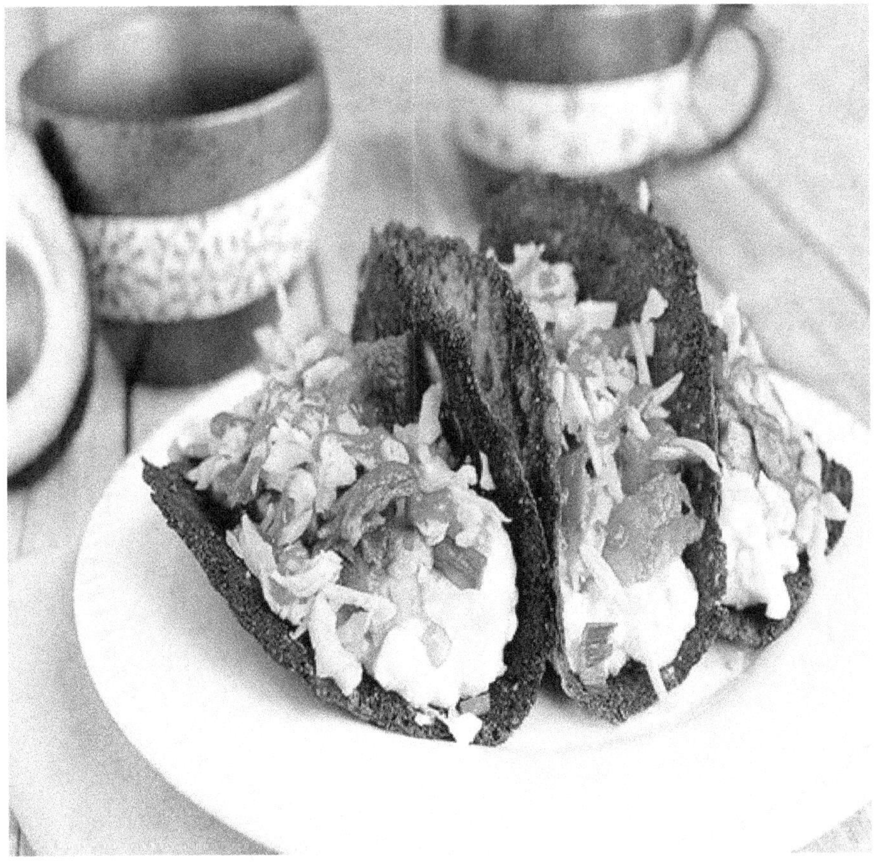

# Flourless Matcha Latte Pancakes

Preparation time: 5 minutes

Cooking time: 5-6 minutes per pancake

Number of servings: 2

Nutritional values per serving: 3 pancakes

Calories – 453, Fat – 38.9 g, Carbohydrate – 12.6 g, Net Carbohydrate – 7.7 g, Protein – 14.6 g

## Ingredients:

- 4 rounded tablespoons unsweetened nut seed butter of your choice
- 2 large eggs
- 2 tablespoons butter + extra to serve
- 4 scoops matcha powder (Perfect Keto MCT)
- ½ cup blueberries (optional)

## Method:

1. Add nut seed butter and matcha powder into a bowl and mix until well incorporated.
2. Add eggs and whisk until well incorporated. You will end up with a batter that is sticky.
3. Place a large nonstick skillet over medium heat. Add about teaspoon of butter. When butter melts, pour enough batter to make 2 inch round pancakes. Make 3-4 pancakes or as many that can fit in the pan.
4. Scatter blueberries over them. Press them lightly on the pancake. When the underside is cooked, flip sides and cook the other side.
5. Serve right away topped with butter.
6. Repeat steps 3-5 and make the remaining pancakes. (**figure. 2**)

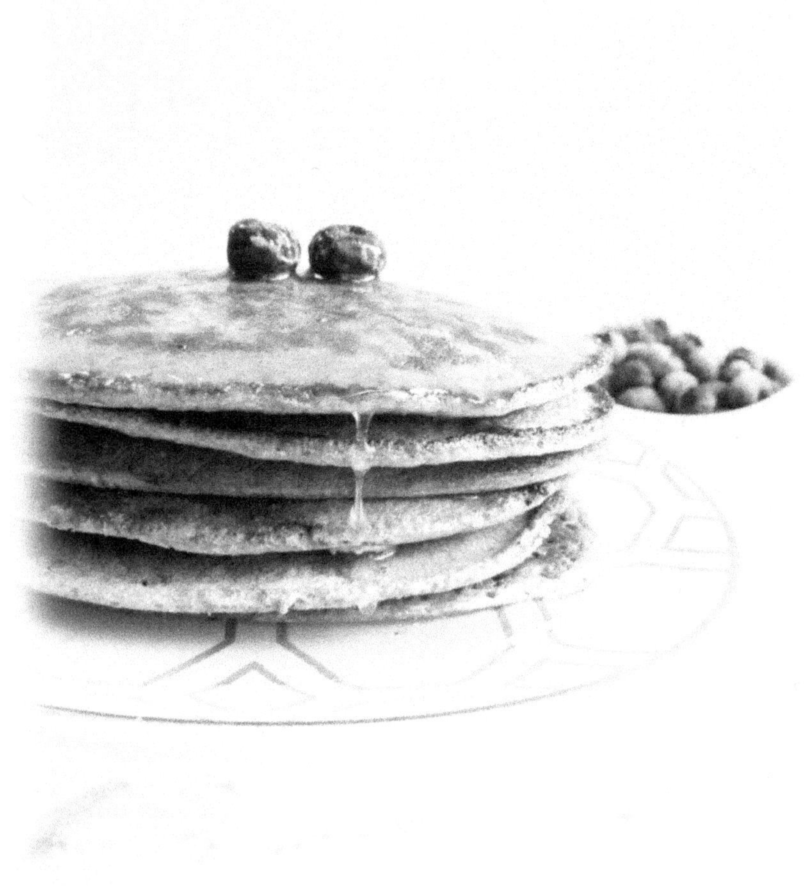

**Figure 2.  Flourless Matcha Latte Pancakes**

# Cheesy Brussels sprouts and Bacon Casserole

Preparation time: 10 minutes

Cooking time: 25 minutes

Number of servings: 3

Nutritional values per serving:

Calories – 325, Fat – 27.3 g, Carbohydrate – 9 g, Net Carbohydrate – 6 g, Protein – 14.2 g

## Ingredients:

- 4 slices bacon, cut into strips
- 1 tablespoon avocado oil
- Avocado oil cooking spray
- ½ tablespoon garlic, minced
- 2 tablespoons cheddar cheese, shredded
- A pinch grated nutmeg
- ½ pound Brussels sprouts, rinsed, pat dried, cut into quarters
- Salt to taste
- Pepper to taste
- ½ small yellow onion, chopped
- ½ cup Parmesan cheese, grated
- 6 tablespoons heavy whipping cream

## Method:

1. Switch on your oven and let it preheat to 375° F.
2. Place a sheet of aluminum foil on a baking sheet. Set aside.
3. Place a pan over medium heat. Add bacon strips and cook until they turn crisp. Remove the bacon with a

slotted spoon and place on a plate lined with paper towels.

4. Add onion and garlic into the same pan and cook in the fat released by the bacon, until onion turns translucent.
5. Add bacon and mix well. Turn off the heat.
6. Meanwhile, add Brussels sprouts, salt, pepper and avocado oil into a bowl and toss well. Spread onto the prepared baking sheet.
7. Place the baking sheet in the oven and bake the Brussels sprouts for about 15 minutes.
8. Spray a casserole dish with cooking spray. Add Brussels sprouts into the casserole dish. Also, add the bacon mixture and mix well.
9. Add cheddar cheese, Parmesan cheese, whipping cream, salt, pepper and nutmeg into a bowl. Whisk well and pour over the Brussels sprouts.
10. Place casserole dish in the oven and bake for 15 minutes. Broil for a few minutes until the top is golden brown.
11. Remove the dish from the oven. Cool for a few minutes and serve. (**figure. 3**)

**Figure 3.   Cheesy Brussels sprouts and Bacon Casserole**

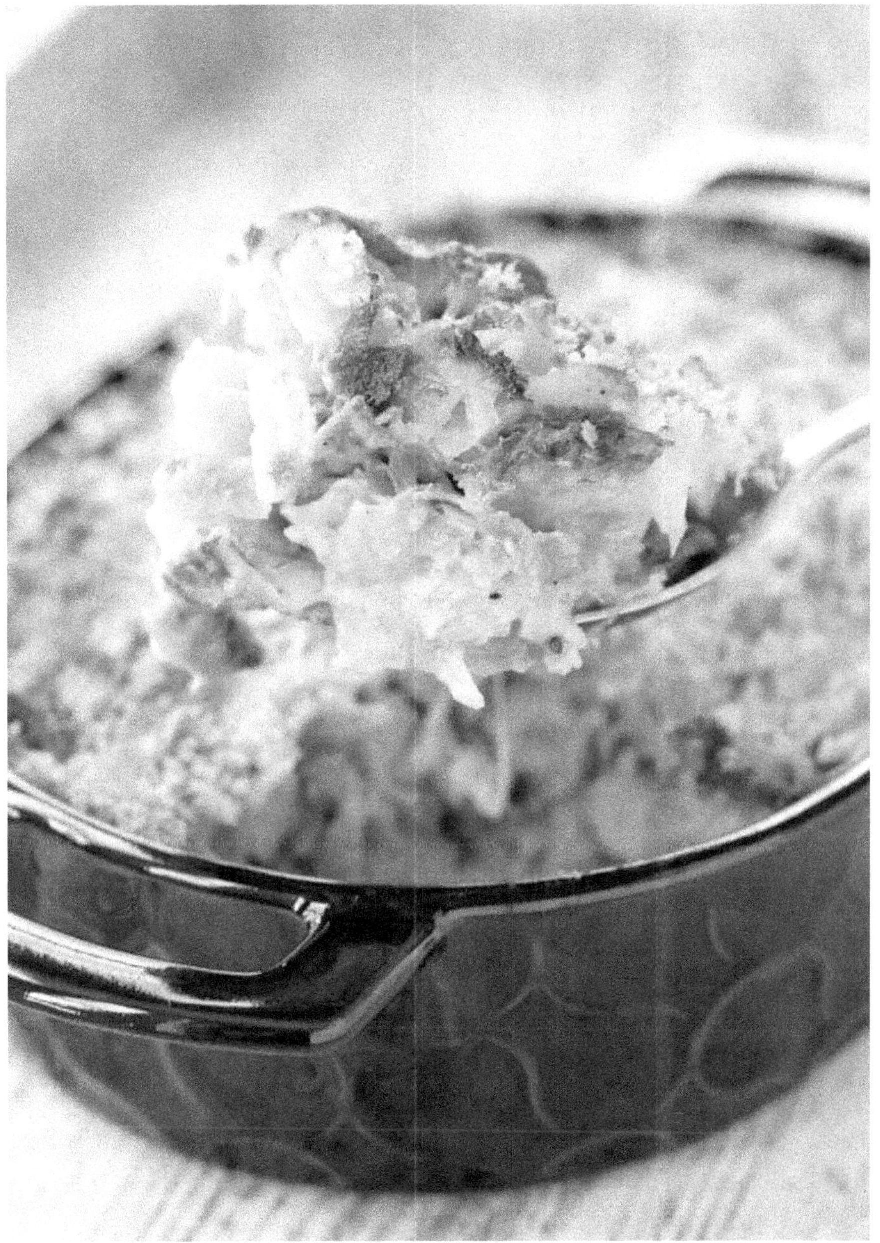

# Caprese Egg Casserole

Preparation time: 5 minutes

Cooking time: 30 minutes

Number of servings: 4

Nutritional values per serving:

Calories – 151, Fat – 11.38 g, Carbohydrate – 2.16 g, Net Carbohydrate – 1.68 g, Protein – 9.8 g

**Ingredients:**

- 1 tablespoon olive oil
- 4 large eggs
- 2 ounces fresh Mozzarella balls
- 1 cup cherry tomatoes, halved or quartered
- 1 tablespoon fresh basil, chopped
- Salt to taste
- Pepper to taste

**Method:**

1. Switch on your oven and let it preheat to 350° F.
2. Place a skillet over medium heat. Add oil. When the oil is heated, add tomatoes and cook until slightly soft. Remove from heat and cool.
3. Whisk eggs in a bowl. Add salt, pepper and basil. Whisk until well combined.
4. Transfer into a casserole dish that is greased with some cooking spray.
5. Scatter tomatoes and Mozzarella balls over the eggs.
6. Place dish in the oven and bake until the eggs are fully set.

7.  Serve hot or warm. **(figure 4.)**

**Figure 4. Caprese Egg Casserole.**

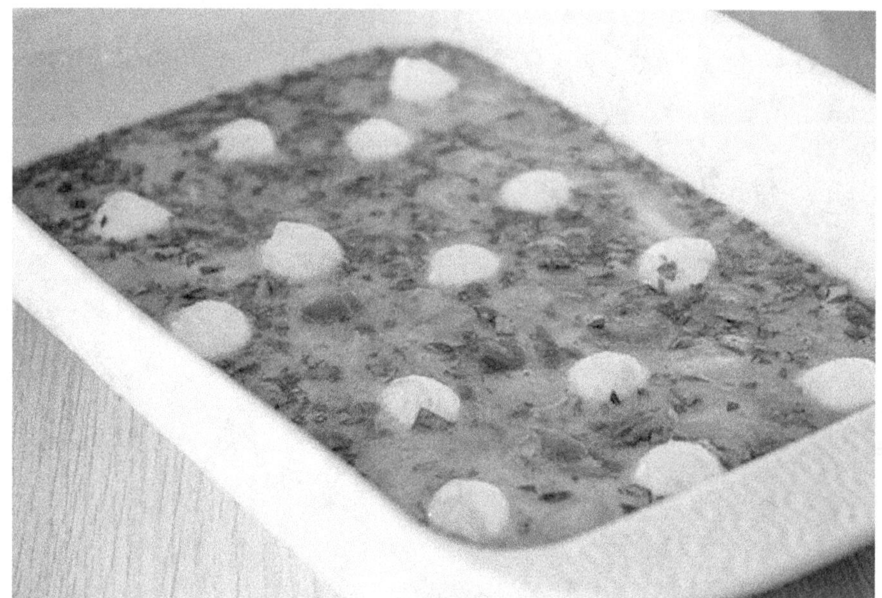

# Chicken Enchilada Bowl

Preparation time: 20 minutes

Cooking time: 30 minutes

Number of servings: 2

Nutritional values per serving: Without cauliflower rice

Calories – 568, Fat – 40.21 g, Carbohydrate – 10.41 g, Net Carbohydrate – 6.14 g, Protein – 38.38 g

**Ingredients:**

- 1 tablespoon coconut oil
- 6 tablespoons red enchilada sauce
- 2 tablespoons chopped onion
- ½ pound chicken thighs, skinless, boneless
- 2 tablespoons water
- 2 ounces canned diced green chilies

For toppings:

- ½ avocado, peeled, pitted, chopped
- 2 tablespoons chopped pickled jalapenos
- 1 small Roma tomato, chopped
- ½ cup cheese, shredded
- ¼ cup sour cream

To serve (optional):

- Cauliflower rice

**Method:**

1. Place a Dutch oven over medium heat. Add oil. When the oil is heated, add chicken thighs and cook until light brown on all the sides.

2. Add enchilada sauce and water and stir.
3. Stir in the onion and green chilies. Lower the heat to low heat and cook until chicken is done.
4. When done, remove chicken with a slotted spoon and place on your countertop.
5. When cool enough to handle, cut into pieces or shred with a pair of forks.
6. Add chicken into the Dutch oven and stir. Cook on low heat for 5-8 minutes.
7. Divide into 2 bowls. Top with the suggested toppings and serve as it is or with cauliflower rice.(**figure. 5**)

Figure 5.  Chicken Enchilada Bowl.

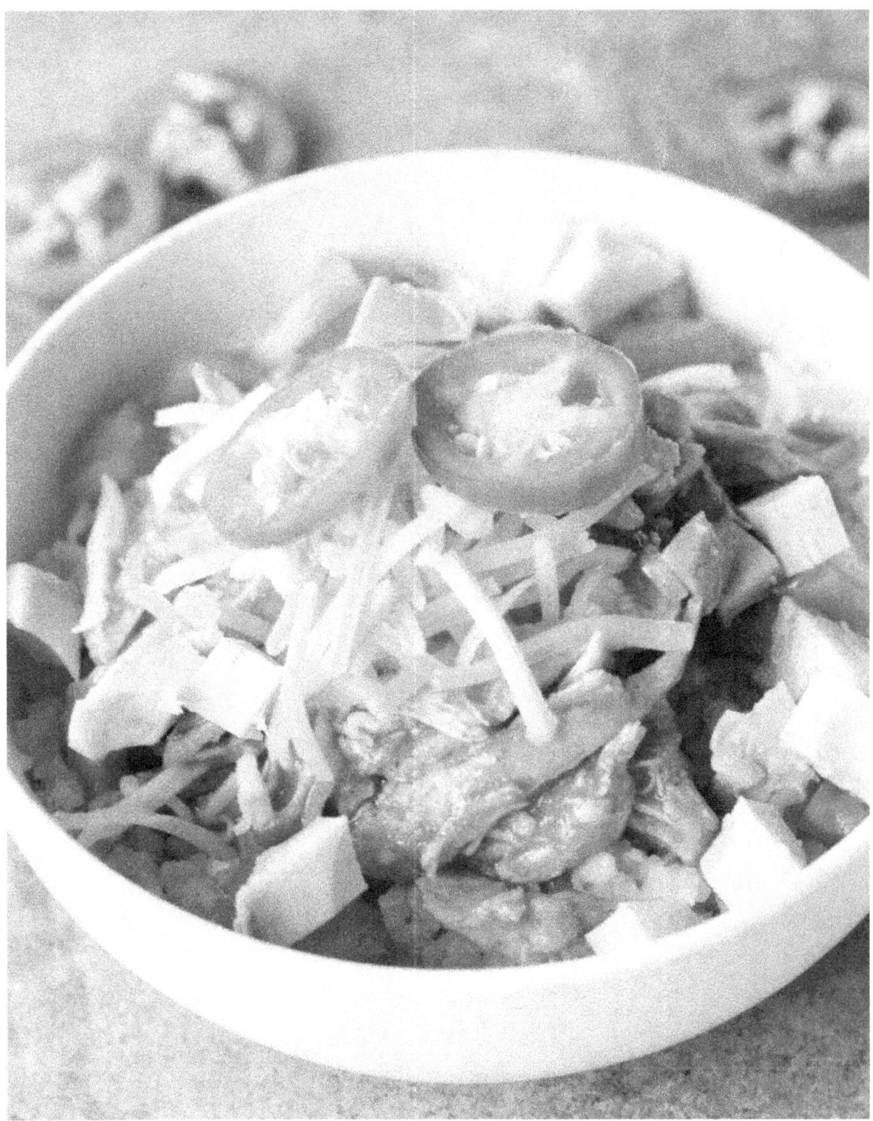

# Broccoli Cheese Soup with Prosciutto

Preparation time: 10 minutes

Cooking time: 30 minutes

Number of servings: 8

Nutritional values per serving:

Calories – 445, Fat – 40 g, Carbohydrate – 6 g, Net Carbohydrate – NA, Protein – 10 g

**Ingredients:**

- 8 cups chicken stock
- 1 onion, chopped
- 2 cups heavy whipping cream
- 2 cups aged Cheddar cheese, grated
- 8 slices prosciutto
- 1 large broccoli, chopped
- 2 cloves garlic, crushed
- 2/3 cup Parmesan cheese, shredded
- 4 tablespoons olive oil
- Salt to taste
- Pine nuts to garnish

**Method:**

1. Place a large pot over medium heat. Add oil. When the oil is heated, add onion and garlic and sauté until onion turns pink.
2. Stir in the broccoli and broth and cook until tender.
3. Turn off the heat. Blend with an immersion blender until creamy.

4.  Place the pot over medium heat. Add cheese, salt and cream and mix well.
5.  Heat until the cheese melts and is well blended in the soup.
6.  Place a pan over medium heat. Add prosciutto and cook until the underside is slightly crisp. Flip sides and cook the other side until slightly crisp.
7.  Ladle soup into soup bowls. Top with prosciutto and pine nuts and serve.(**fig. 6**)

**Figure 6. Broccoli Cheese Soup with Prosciutto**

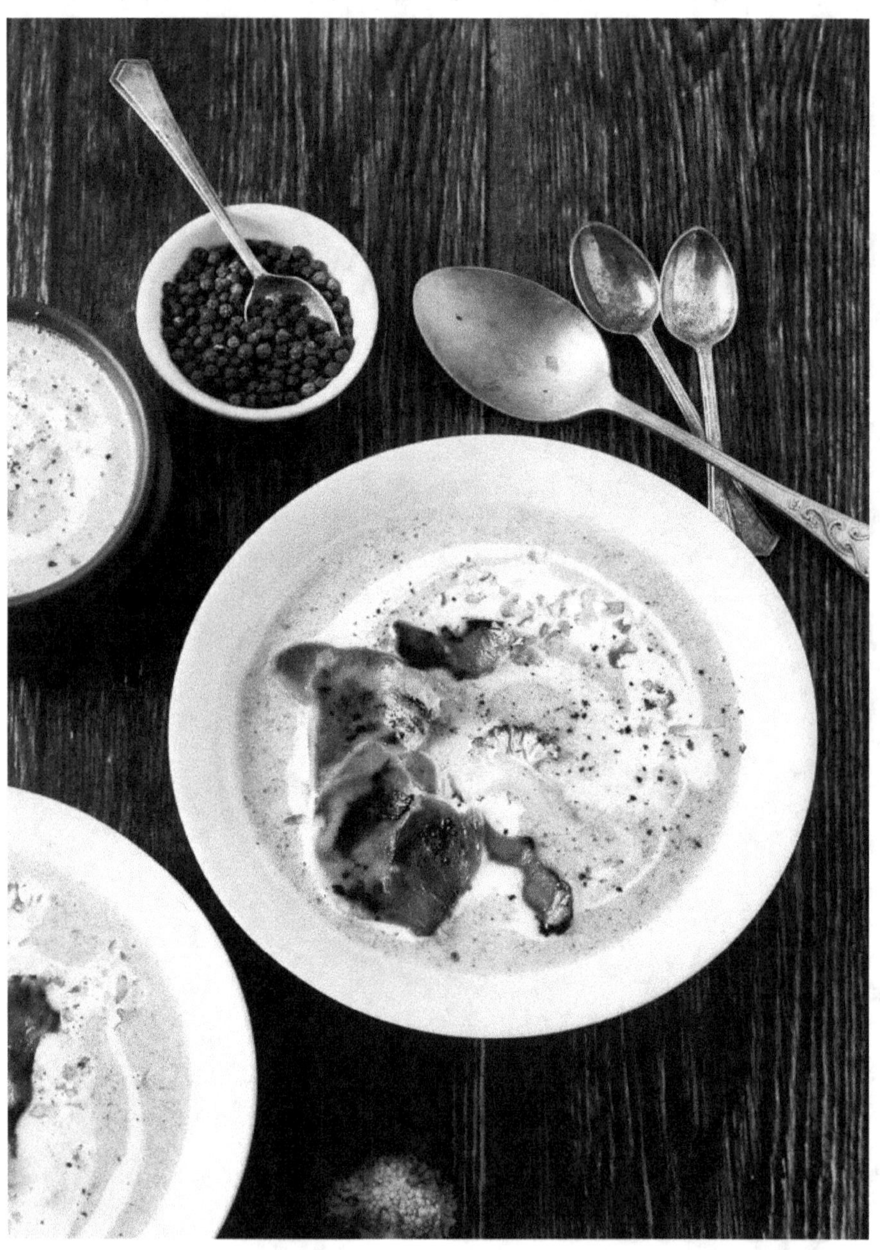

# Tomato and Feta Soup

Preparation time: 8 minutes

Cooking time: 30 minutes

Number of servings: 12

Nutritional values per serving:

Calories – 170, Fat – 13 g, Carbohydrate – 10 g, Net Carbohydrate – 8 g, Protein – 4 g

## Ingredients:

- 4 tablespoons butter or olive oil
- 4 cloves garlic, minced
- Black pepper powder to taste
- 1 teaspoon dried oregano
- 2 tablespoons tomato paste (optional)
- 2 teaspoons erythritol (optional)
- 2/3 cup Feta cheese, crumbled
- ½ cup onion, chopped
- 1 teaspoon salt
- 2 teaspoons pesto sauce (optional)
- 2 teaspoons dried basil
- 20 tomatoes, peeled, deseeded, chopped or 4 cans (14.5 ounces each) peeled tomatoes
- 6 cups water

## Method:

1. Place a large soup pot over medium heat. Add butter. When butter melts, add onion and sauté until translucent.

2.  Add garlic and sauté until aromatic.
3.  Stir in the tomatoes, oregano, tomatoes, tomato paste, salt, pepper, basil, oregano and water.
4.  When it begins to boil, lower the heat and add erythritol. Cover and cook until tomatoes are soft.
5.  Blend with an immersion blender until creamy.
6.  Stir in the heavy cream and Feta cheese. Mix well. Turn off the heat.
7.  Taste and adjust the seasoning if necessary.
8.  Ladle into soup bowls. Serve hot or warm.(**figure. 7**)

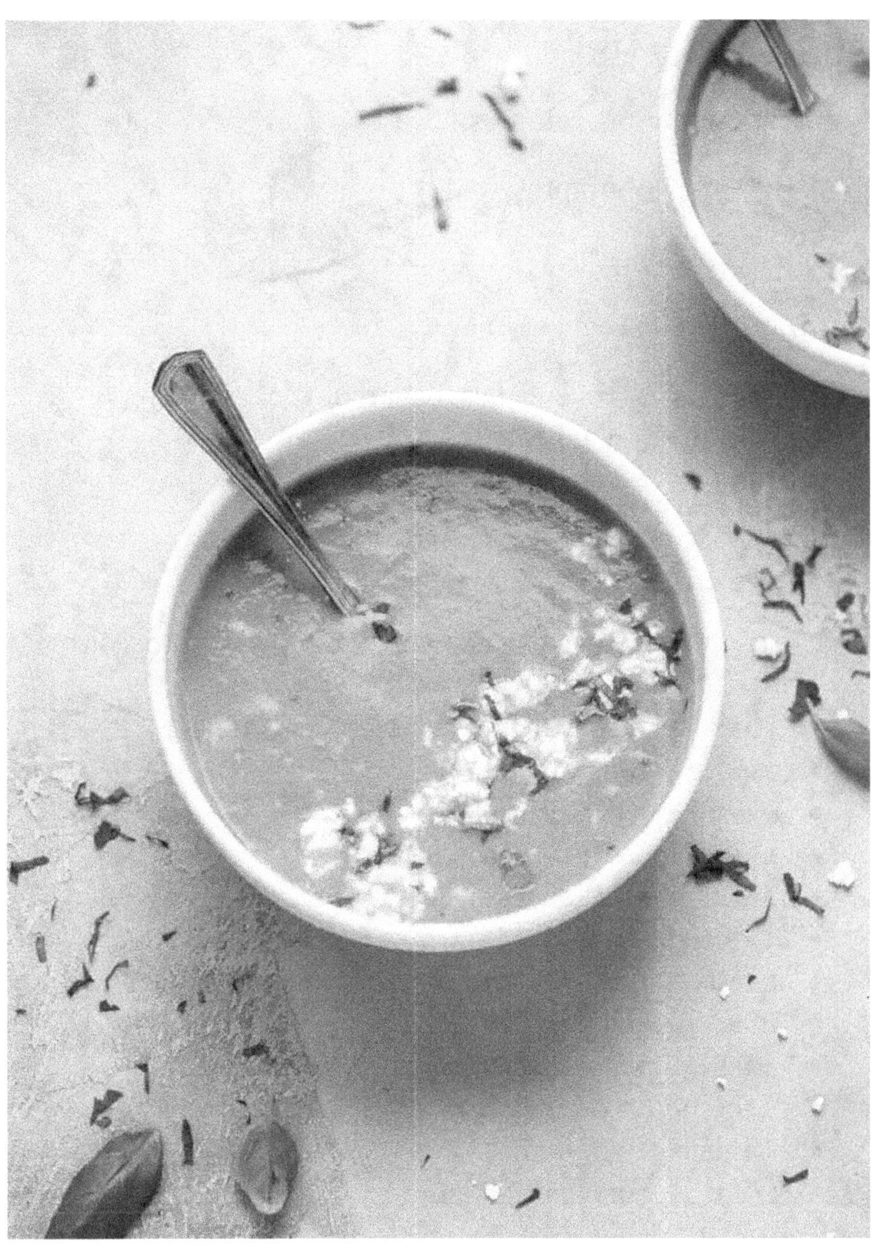

**Figure 7.  Tomato and Feta Soup**

# Chicken Pot Pie

Preparation time: 15 minutes

Cooking time: 20 minutes

Number of servings:

Nutritional values per serving:

Calories – 297, Fat – 17 g, Carbohydrate – 5.3 g, Net Carbohydrate – 3.3 g, Protein – 11.6 g

**Ingredients:**

For chicken pot pie filling:

- ¼ cup mixed vegetables (cauliflower, broccoli and carrot)
- Himalayan pink salt to taste
- 1 clove garlic, minced
- ½ cup chicken broth
- 1/8 teaspoon dried rosemary
- 1 ¼ cups chicken, cooked, chopped
- 1 tablespoon butter
- 2 tablespoons chopped onion
- Black pepper powder to taste
- 6 tablespoons heavy whipping cream
- 2 teaspoons poultry seasoning
- A pinch dried thyme
- 1/8 teaspoon xanthan gum

For the crust:

- 3 tablespoons coconut flour
- 7 teaspoons butter, melted, cooled
- 1 tablespoon full fat sour cream
- 1/8 teaspoon salt

- 2/3 cup sharp Cheddar cheese or Mozzarella cheese, shredded

**Method:**

1. Place a skillet over medium heat.
2. Place an ovenproof skillet over medium heat. Add butter. When butter melts, add onion and sauté for a couple of minutes.
3. Add mixed vegetables, salt, pepper and garlic and sauté for another 2 minutes.
4. Stir in the whipping cream seasoning, dried herbs and broth.
5. Dust the xanthan gum on top and stir. Cover and cook until thick.
6. Stir in the chicken.
7. To make crust: Add melted butter, salt, eggs and sour cream into a bowl and mix until well combined.
8. Stir in the coconut flour and baking powder and mix until well incorporated.
9. Add cheese and mix well.
10. Drop teaspoonfuls of batter at different spots on the potpie.
11. Switch on your oven and let it preheat to 400° F.
12. Place rack in the upper part of the oven. Place skillet on the rack.
13. Broil for a few minutes until brown on top.(**figure. 8**)

**Figure 8.  Chicken Pot Pie.**

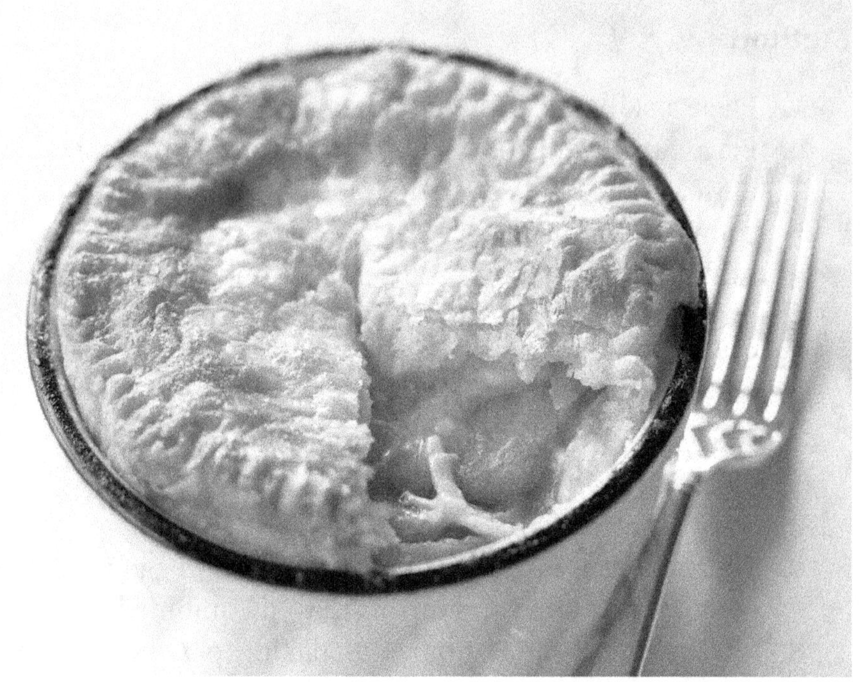

# Chicken & Goat Cheese Skillet

Preparation time: 10 minutes

Cooking time: 15 minutes

Number of servings: 4

Nutritional values per serving: 1-½ cups (without cauliflower rice)

Calories – 251, Fat – 11 g, Carbohydrate – 8 g, Net Carbohydrate – 5 g, Protein – 29 g

**Ingredients:**

- 1 pound chicken breast, skinless, boneless, cut into 1 inch pieces
- ¼ teaspoon pepper powder
- 2 cups fresh asparagus (cut into 1 inch pieces)
- 6 plum tomatoes, chopped
- ¾ cup herbed fresh goat's cheese, crumbled
- ½ teaspoon salt or to taste
- 4 teaspoons olive oil
- 2 cloves garlic, minced
- 6 tablespoons 2% milk
- Cauliflower rice to serve (optional)

**Method:**

1. Season chicken with salt and pepper.
2. Place a large skillet over medium high heat. Add oil. When the oil is heated, add chicken and cook until it is not pink anymore. Remove into a bowl and keep it warm.

3. Stir in the asparagus into the skillet and cook for a
   minute. Stir in asparagus and cook until fragrant.
4. Add rest of the ingredients and cook until cheese melts.
5. Add chicken and stir.
6. Serve over cauliflower rice.

Figure 9.  Chicken & Goat Cheese Skillet.

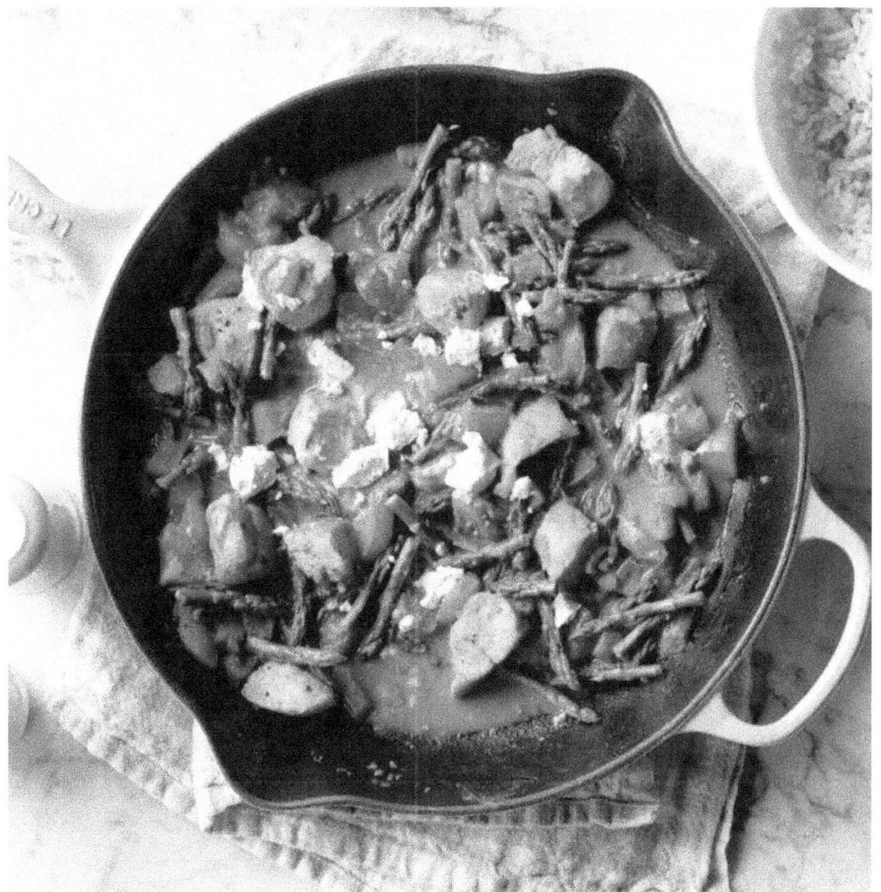

# Big Mac Salad

Preparation time: 10 minutes

Cooking time: 10 minutes

Number of servings: 3

Nutritional values per serving:

Calories – 368, Fat – 31 g, Carbohydrate – 3 g, Net Carbohydrate – 2 g, Protein – 18 g

**Ingredients:**

For salad:

- ½ pound ground beef
- Black pepper powder to taste
- Salt to taste
- 4 ounces Romaine lettuce
- 6 tablespoons Cheddar cheese, shredded
- ½ cup tomatoes, chopped
- ¼ cup pickles (chopped)

For dressing:

- ¼ cup keto friendly mayonnaise
- 1 teaspoon mustard
- ¼ teaspoon smoked paprika
- 1 tablespoon pickles, chopped
- ½ teaspoon white vinegar
- ¾ tablespoon powdered erythritol

**Method:**

1. Place a skillet over high heat. Add beef, salt and pepper. Cook until brown. Break it simultaneously as it cooks.

2. Add all the ingredients of dressing into a blender and blend until smooth. Add water to dilute the dressing if desired.
3. Transfer into a bowl and chill until use.
4. Add rest of the salad ingredients into a bowl and toss well. Add browned beef and toss again.
5. Add dressing. Mix well.
6. Divide into 3 plates and serve.(**figure. 10**)

# Figure 10.   Big Mac Salad

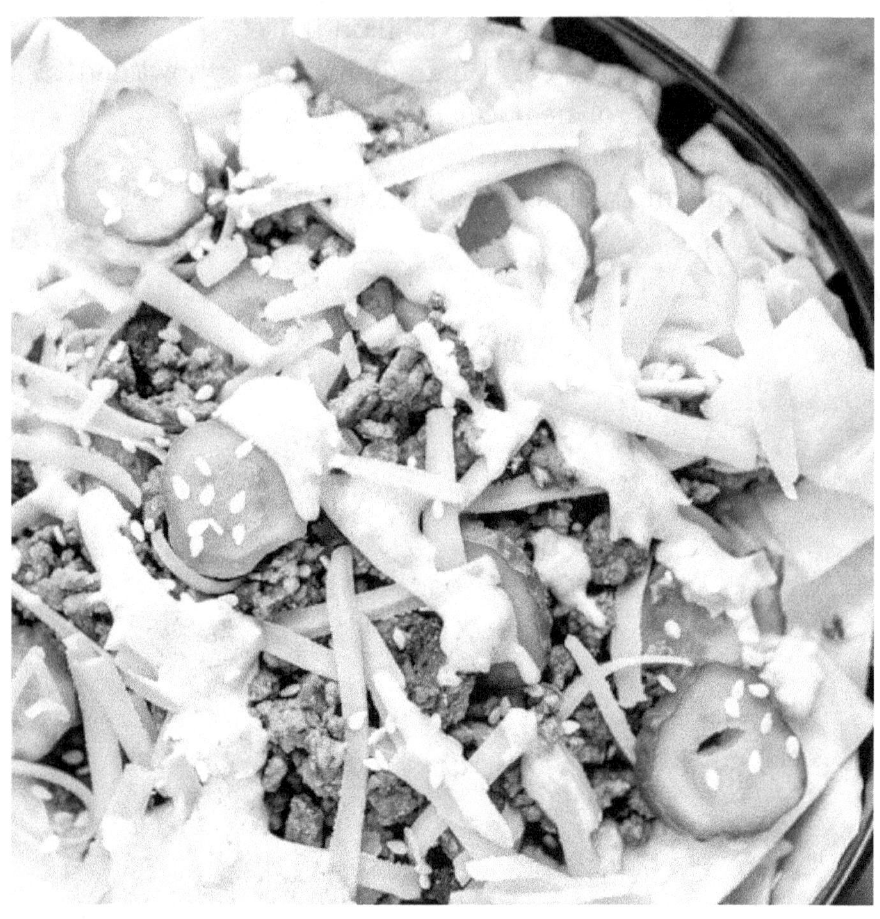

# Loaded Cauliflower Mash Bake

Preparation time: 10 minutes

Cooking time: 20 minutes

Number of servings: 8

Nutritional values per serving:

Calories – 112, Fat – 5.5 g, Carbohydrate – 10 g, Net Carbohydrate – 6 g, Protein – 1.5 g

## Ingredients:

- 8 slices center cut bacon, cooked, crumbled
- 6 cloves crushed garlic
- 2 tablespoons whipped butter
- Freshly ground black pepper to taste
- ½ cup low fat Cheddar cheese, shredded
- 12 cups (about 48 ounces) cauliflower florets
- 2/3 cup buttermilk
- 1 ½ teaspoons Kosher salt
- ¼ cup fresh chives, minced, divided

## Method:

1. Place a pot of water over high heat. When it begins to boil, add cauliflower and garlic and cook until soft.
2. Drain and add it back into the pot. Add butter, buttermilk, pepper and salt and blend with an immersion blender until smooth. Add half the chives and stir.
3. Divide into 8 small casserole dishes. Sprinkle Cheddar cheese and bacon.
4. Switch on your oven and let it preheat to 350° F.
5. Place dishes in the oven and cook until cheese melts. Bake in batches if necessary.

6.  Garnish with remaining chives and serve.(**figure.** 11)

**Figure 11. Loaded Cauliflower Mash Bake.**

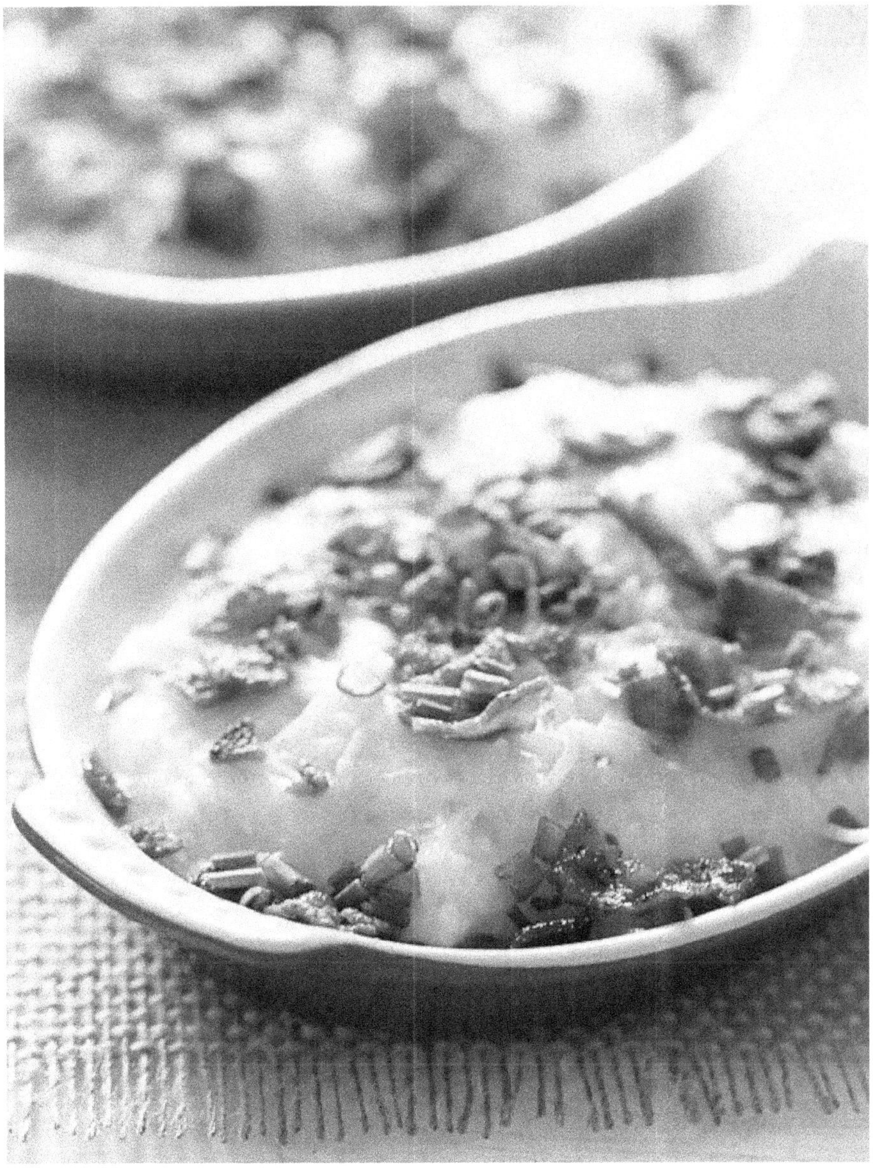

# Tomato Mozzarella and Arugula Tower

Preparation time: 10 minutes

Cooking time: 0 minutes

Number of servings: 4

Nutritional values per serving:

Calories – 276.6, Fat – 23 g, Carbohydrate – 9.2 g, Net Carbohydrate – 7.3 g, Protein – 12.2 g

## Ingredients:

- ½ cup basil, chopped
- 4 tablespoons olive oil
- 4 medium ripe tomatoes
- 4 cups arugula
- 2 tablespoons balsamic vinegar
- Kosher salt to taste
- Fresh pepper to taste
- 6 ounces part skim Mozzarella cheese, cut into 12 slices

## Method:

1. Add basil, vinegar, oil, salt and pepper into a small blender and blend until smooth.
2. Cut a slice off from the top as well as bottom of each of the tomatoes and discard it.
3. Make 3 equal slices of each tomato.
4. Take 4 serving plates. Scatter ¾ cup arugula on each plate. Place 1 tomato (3 slices) in each plate.
5. Layer with Mozzarella followed by ¼ cup arugula (make a tower) in each plate.

6. Sprinkle pepper. Trickle 1-tablespoon oil and ½ tablespoon vinegar on each tower and serve.(**figure. 12**)

Figure 12.   Tomato Mozzarella and Arugula Tower.

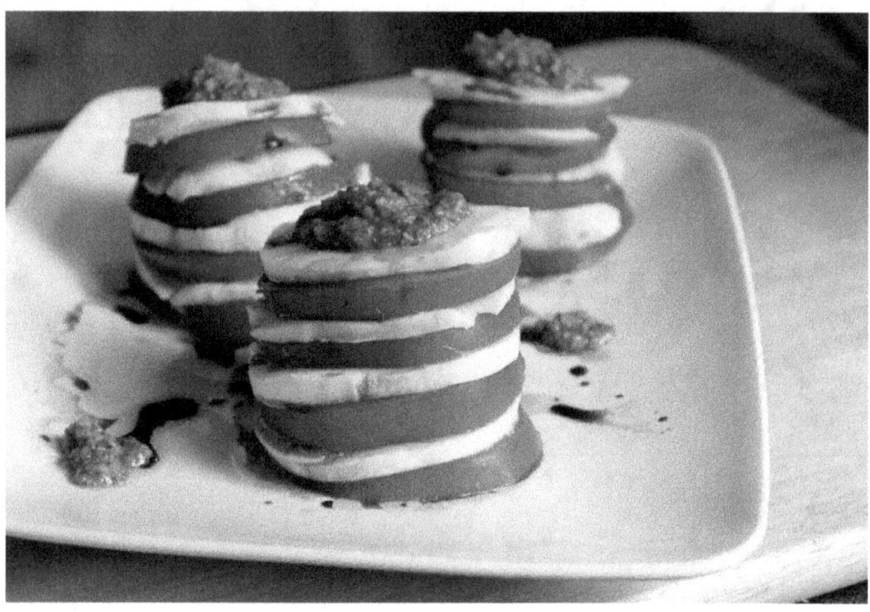

# Zucchini Beef Sauté

Preparation time: 5 minutes

Cooking time: 10 minutes

Number of servings: 4

Nutritional values per serving:

Calories – 500, Fat – 40 g, Carbohydrate – 5 g, Net Carbohydrate – 1 g, Protein – 31 g

**Ingredients:**

- 20 ounces beef, cut into 1 to 2 inch long thin strips
- ½ cup cilantro, chopped
- 4 tablespoons tamari sauce or coconut aminos
- 2 zucchinis, cut into 1-2 inch long thin strips
- 6 cloves garlic, chopped or minced
- 4 tablespoons avocado oil or coconut oil or olive oil

**Method:**

1. Place a pan over high heat. Add oil. When the oil is heated, add beef and cook until brown on both the sides.
2. Add zucchini and cook until tender.
3. Add tamari, cilantro and garlic. Cook for a couple of minutes and serve.

**Figure 13.  Zucchini Beef Saute**

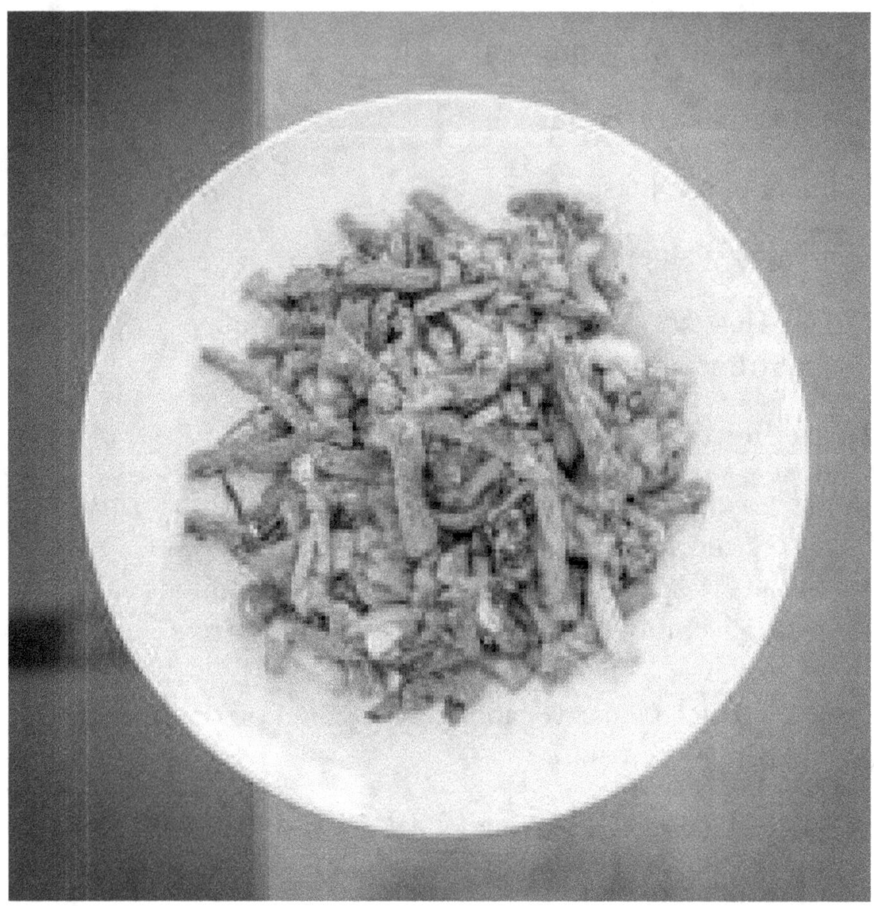

# Greek Meatballs Salad

Preparation time: 10 minutes

Cooking time: 20 minutes

Number of servings: 8

Nutritional values per serving:

Calories – 399, Fat – 36 g, Carbohydrate – 2 g, Net Carbohydrate – NA, Protein – 20 g

**Ingredients:**

<u>For meatballs:</u>

- 2 pounds ground lamb or beef
- ½ cup mint, finely chopped
- Salt to taste
- Pepper powder to taste
- 4 teaspoons dried oregano
- 4 cloves garlic, minced
- Olive oil to fry, as required

<u>For salad:</u>

- 2 tomatoes, cut into wedges
- 2 lemons, cut into wedges
- Lettuce leaves to serve
- ½ cup flat leaf parsley, chopped

**Method:**

1. Switch on your oven and let it preheat to 35 0° F.
2. Add all the ingredients of meatballs into a bowl and mix until well combined. Make small portions and shape into balls.

3.  Place a large pan over medium heat. Add some oil. When the oil is heated, place some meatballs and cook until brown on all the sides. Transfer onto a baking sheet lined with parchment paper. Cook in batches.
4.  Place baking sheet in the oven and bake for 10 minutes or until well cooked inside.
5.  Mix together lettuce and tomato in a bowl. Divide the salad into 8 serving plates.
6.  Top with meatballs and serve garnished with parsley and lemon wedges.(**fig. 14**)

# Figure 14.  Greek Meatballs Salad

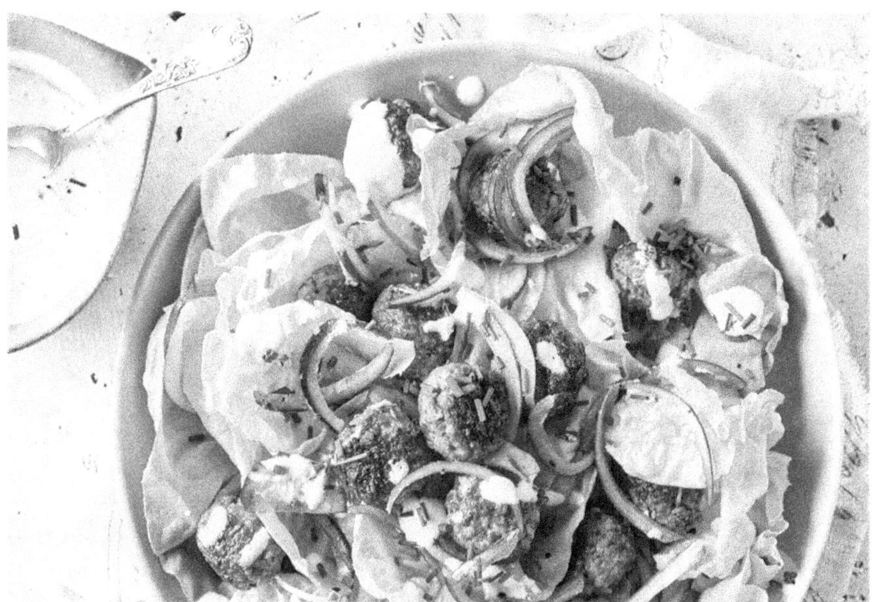

# Fat Bomb Pork Chops

Preparation time: 12-15 minutes

Cooking time: 30 minutes

Number of servings: 6

Nutritional values per serving:

Calories – 1121, Fat – 104 g, Carbohydrate – 9 g, Net Carbohydrate – 8 g, Protein – 35 g

## Ingredients:

- 2 medium onions, sliced
- 1 cup oil
- 2 teaspoons garlic powder
- 2 cups keto friendly mayonnaise
- 2 packages (8 ounces each) brown mushrooms, sliced
- 6 medium pork chops, boneless
- 2 teaspoons ground nutmeg
- 2 tablespoons balsamic vinegar

## Method:

1. Place a large skillet over medium heat. Add oil. When the oil is heated, add onion and mushroom and sauté until slightly tender.
2. Transfer into a bowl. Place pork chops in the pan. Sprinkle garlic powder and nutmeg over it. Cook until brown all over and cooked as per your liking.
3. Remove pork with a slotted spoon and set aside.
4. When the onion mixture in the skillet cools, add mayonnaise and vinegar and mix until well incorporated.
5. Place chops on serving plates. Spoon sauce mixture on top and serve.(**figure. 15**)

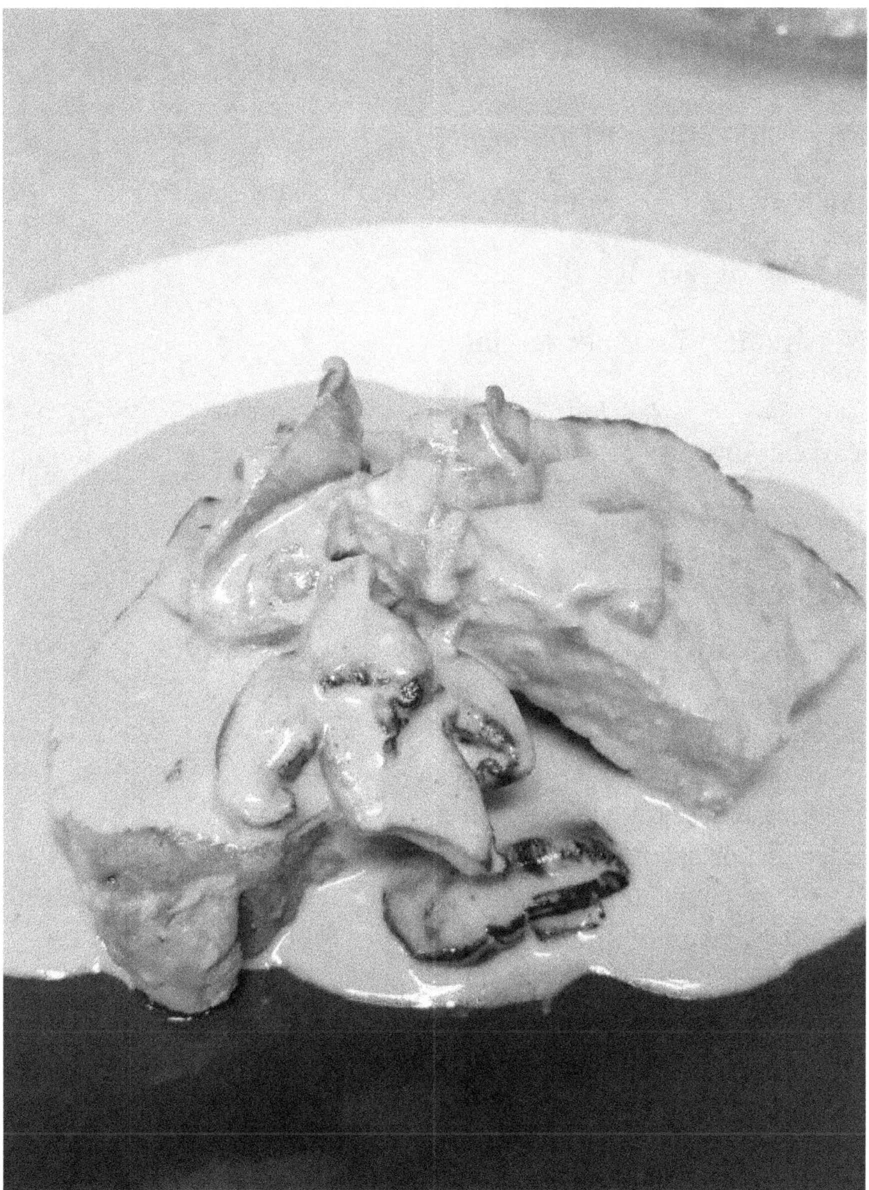

Figure 15.  Fat Bomb Pork Chops.

# Creamy Pork Chops

Preparation time: 10 minutes

Cooking time: 20 minutes

Number of servings: 8

Nutritional values per serving:

Calories – 497, Fat – 35 g, Carbohydrate – 7 g, Net Carbohydrate – 6 g, Protein – 32 g

**Ingredients:**

For pork chops:

- 4 tablespoons butter
- 8 pork chops, boneless

For breading mixture:

- 1 teaspoon garlic powder
- 2 teaspoons Italian seasoning
- 2/3 cup blanched almond flour
- 1 teaspoon onion powder
- Salt to taste
- Freshly ground black pepper to taste

For sauce:

- 4 tablespoons butter
- 1 cup parmesan cheese
- 2 teaspoons fresh lemon juice
- 1 cup heavy cream
- 8 sprigs fresh thyme (leaves only)
- 4 cloves garlic, minced

- 1 cup dry white wine
- 1 cup chicken stock
- 2 teaspoons Italian seasoning

**Method:**

1. Add all the ingredients of breading mixture into a shallow bowl and stir.
2. Coat the chops with breading mixture.
3. Place a large skillet over medium high heat. Add butter. When butter melts, place pork chops and cooks for 3-4 minutes. Flip sides and reduce the heat to medium heat. Cook the other side for 3-4 minutes. Cook in batches if required.
4. Remove with a slotted spoon and place on a plate. Cover and set aside.
5. To make sauce: Add 4 tablespoons butter into the same skillet. When butter melts, add garlic and cook until aromatic.
6. Stir in the wine, stock, cream and lemon juice. When it begins to boil, reduce the heat to low heat and simmer for 3-4 minutes.
7. Stir in Italian seasoning, Parmesan cheese, salt, pepper and thyme. Mix well and simmer for 3-4 minutes. Taste and adjust the seasoning if necessary.
8. Add pork chops back into the skillet. Coat it well with the sauce. Heat thoroughly and serve.(**figure. 16**)

**Figure 16.  Creamy Pork Chops.**

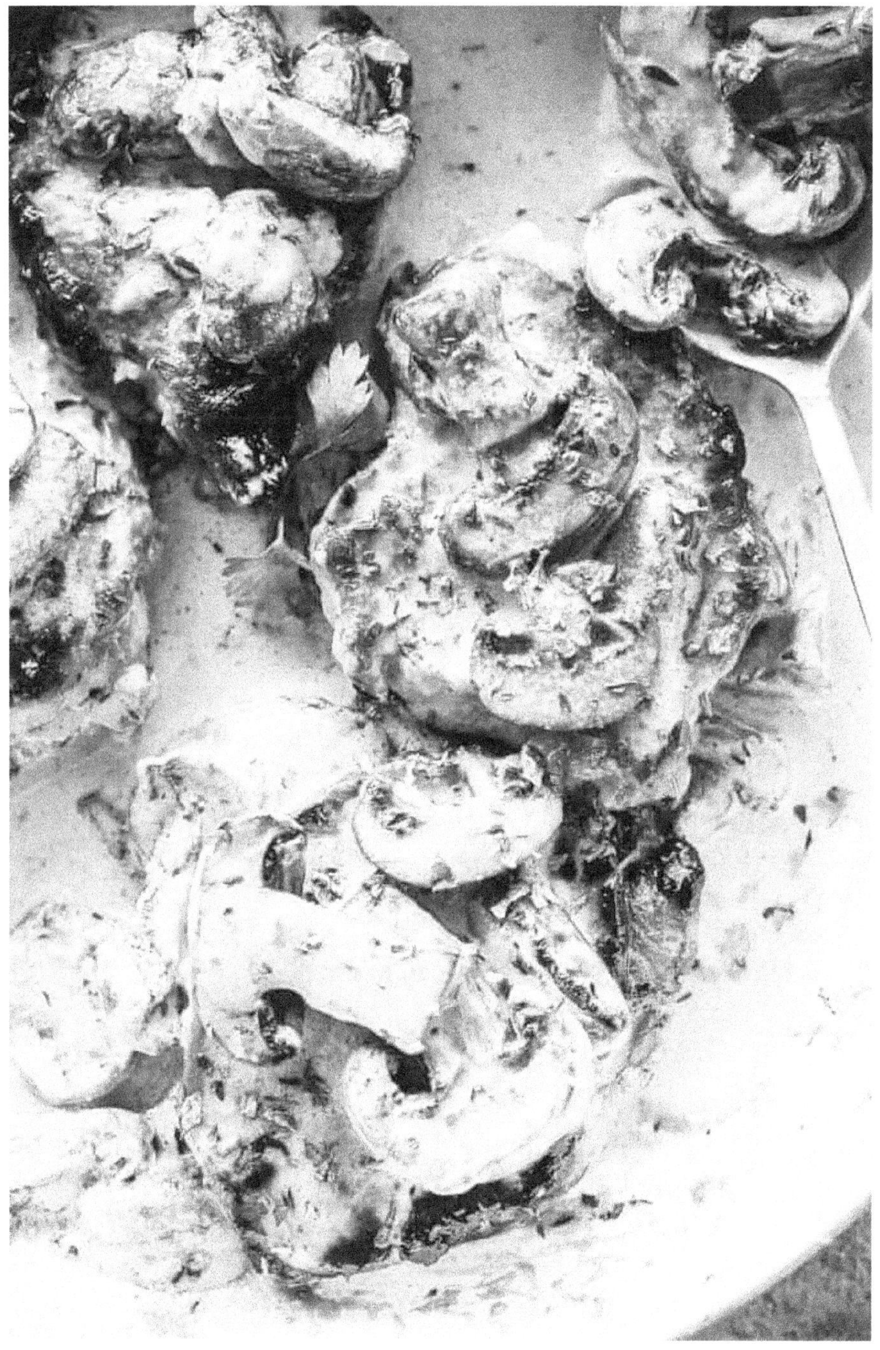

# Bacon Parmesan Spaghetti Squash

Preparation time: 5 minutes

Cooking time: 50-60 minutes

Number of servings: 3

Nutritional values per serving:

Calories – 109, Fat – 7 g, Carbohydrate – 5.3 g, Net Carbohydrate – 4.3 g, Protein – 6 g

**Ingredients:**

- 2 slices center cut bacon, sliced
- Kosher salt to taste
- ¼ cup Parmigiano Reggiano cheese, grated
- 1 small spaghetti squash (you should get 1 ½ cups cooked spaghetti so choose accordingly), halved lengthwise, deseeded
- 2 teaspoons extra-virgin olive oil
- Freshly ground black pepper to taste

**Method:**

1. Place a skillet over medium heat. Place bacon strips and remove when crisp onto a plate lined with paper towels.
2. Switch on your oven and let it preheat to 35 0° F.
3. Place a sheet of aluminum foil on a baking sheet.
4. Sprinkle salt and pepper on the cut side of the spaghetti. Place on the baking sheet with the cut side facing down.
5. Place baking sheet in the oven and bake for 40-50 minutes or until cooked through.

6.  Remove from the oven and let it cool for a while. When
    cool enough to handle, shred with a pair of forks and
    add into a bowl. Add oil, bacon and Parmesan and mix
    well.
7.  Serve.(**figure. 17**)

**Figure 17.  Bacon Parmesan Spaghetti Squash**

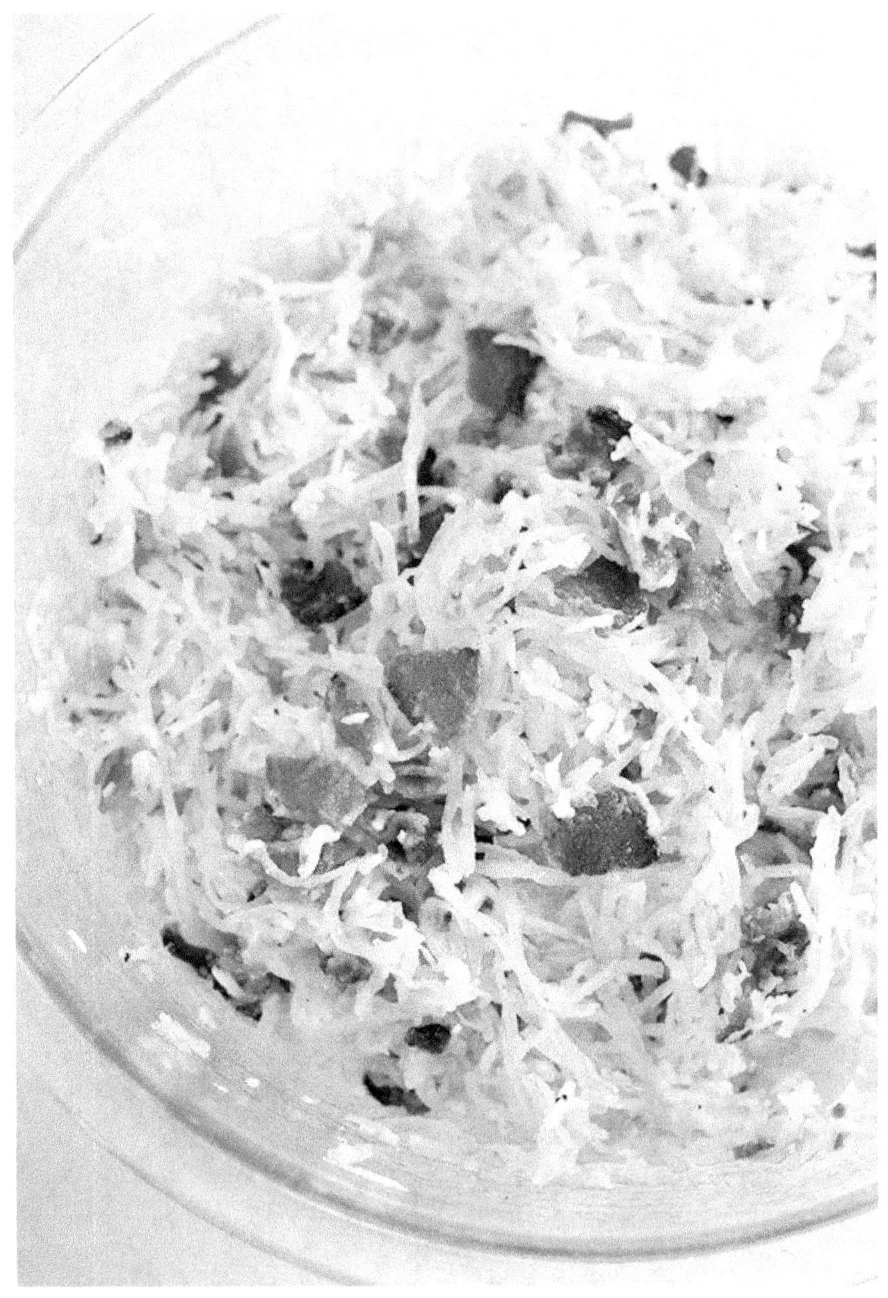

# California Spicy Crab Stuffed Avocado

Preparation time: 10 minutes

Cooking time: 10 minutes

Number of servings: 4

Nutritional values per serving:

Calories – 194, Fat – 13 g, Carbohydrate – 7 g, Net Carbohydrate – 3 g, Protein – 12 g

**Ingredients:**

- 4 tablespoons keto friendly mayonnaise
- 2 teaspoons chopped chives
- ½ cup cucumber, peeled, chopped
- 1 teaspoon furikake seasoning or sesame seeds
- 4 teaspoons sriracha + extra to serve
- 8 ounces lump crab meat
- 2 small Hass avocados, halved
- 4 teaspoons tamari

**Method:**

1. Add sriracha, mayonnaise and chives into a bowl and stir.
2. Stir in crabmeat, cucumber and chives.
3. Peel the avocado and remove the seed. Remove a little of the avocado with a spoon.
4. Fill the avocado cases with crab mixture.
5. Sprinkle furikake and trickle tamari on top and serve.(**figure. 18**)

# Figure 18.  California Spicy Stuffed Avocado

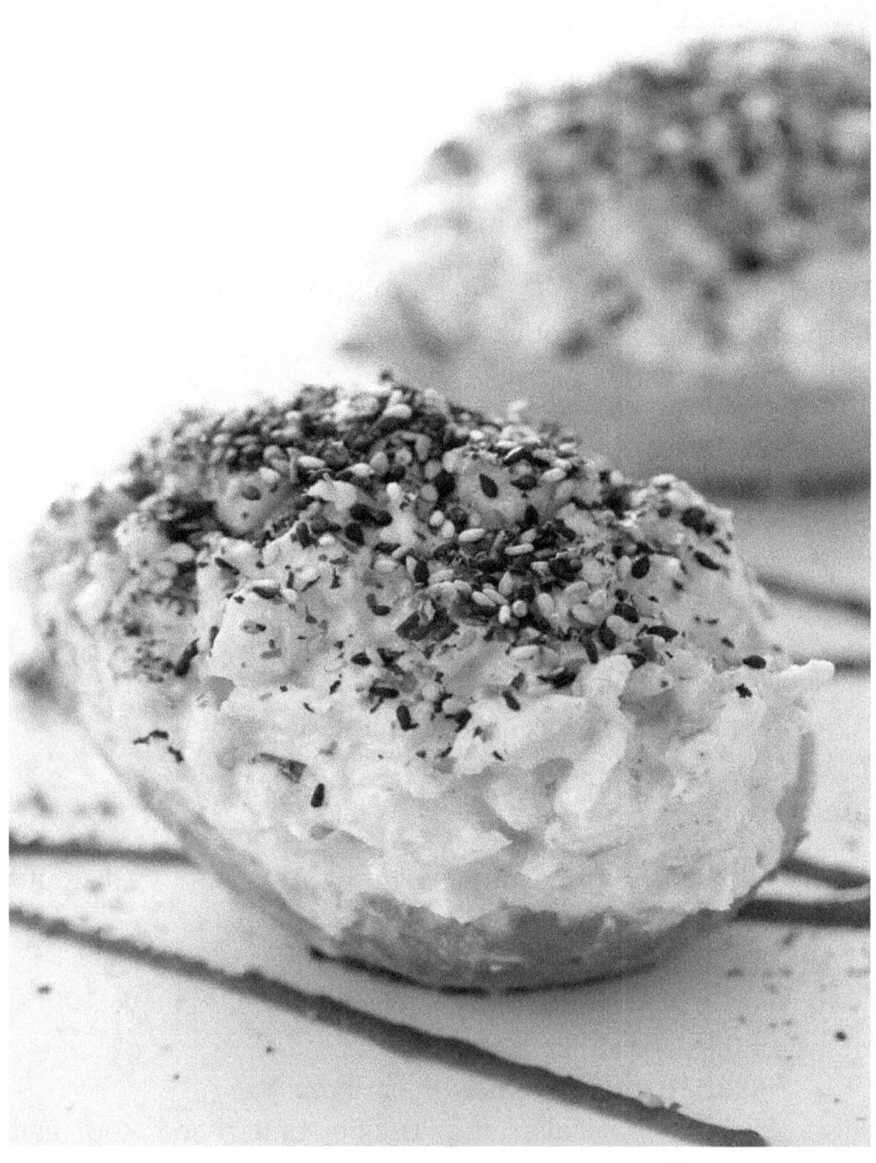

# Raw Chocolate Cheesecake

Preparation time: 6-8 hours

Chilling time: 2-3 hours

Number of servings: 8

Nutritional values per serving:

Calories – 379, Fat – 15.3 g, Carbohydrate – 13 g, Net Carbohydrate – 9.6 g, Protein – 8.9 g

**Ingredients:**

For crust:

- ½ cup walnuts
- 2 tablespoons virgin coconut oil
- 1/8 teaspoon sea salt
- 2 1/3 ounces almond flour
- ½ teaspoon espresso powder (optional)

For filling:

- 1 ½ cups raw cashews, soaked in water for 6-8 hours
- 3 ½ tablespoons virgin coconut oil
- ¼ cup cacao powder
- ¼ cup confectioners' swerve or powdered erythritol
- 3 ounces canned full fat coconut milk
- ½ tablespoon vanilla extract, unsweetened
- 1 ½ tablespoons lemon juice

For topping (ganache):

- 1.5 ounces 100% dark chocolate, divided
- Stevia drops to taste
- 3 tablespoons coconut milk

**Method:**

1. To make crust: Add walnuts, coconut oil, sea salt, almond flour and espresso powder into a food processor bowl and process until crumbly in texture.
2. Transfer into a 6-inch springform pan. Press it well onto the bottom of the pan.
3. To make filling: Add cashews, coconut oil, cacao powder, swerve, coconut milk, vanilla and lemon juice into the food processor and process until very smooth and creamy. Spoon over the crust. Spread it evenly.
4. Place the pan in the freezer and let it freeze for 2 hours.
5. To make ganache: Add coconut milk into a saucepan. Place saucepan over medium heat. When it begins to boil, turn off the heat.
6. Place 1 ounce chocolate in a bowl. Transfer the coconut milk into the bowl of chocolate.
7. Add sweetener and stir until well combined.
8. Spoon the ganache over the topping. Spread it evenly. Sprinkle remaining chocolate.
9. Place pan in the freezer for an hour.
10. Slice and serve. (**figure. 19**)

# Figure 19.  Raw Chocolate Cheescake

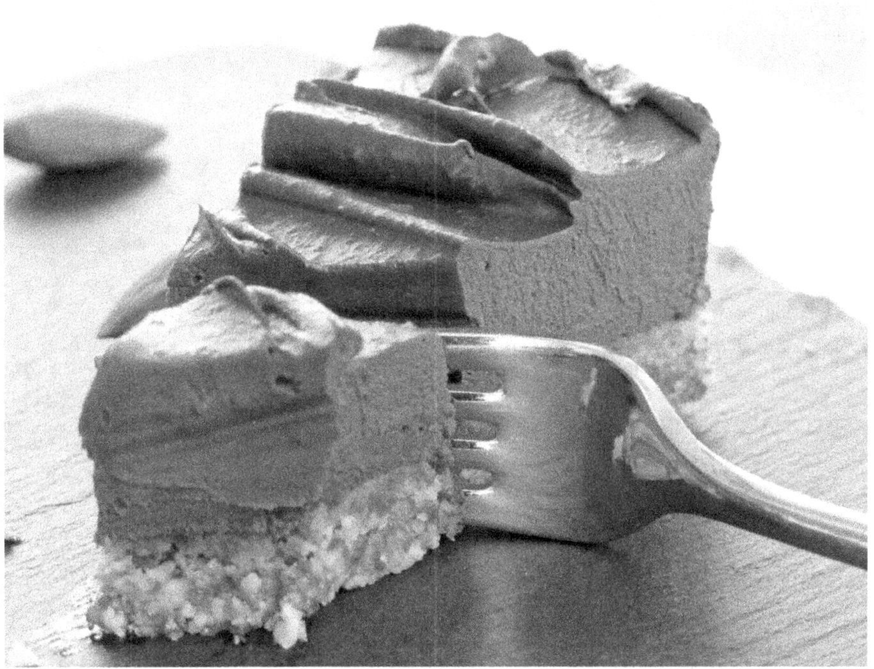

# Keto Chocolate Muffins

Preparation time: minutes

Cooking time: minutes

Number of servings: 6

Nutritional values per serving:

Calories – 115, Fat – 10 g, Carbohydrate – 3.8 g, Net Carbohydrate – 1.4 g, Protein – 4 g

**Ingredients:**

- ½ cup natural creamy almond butter
- 1 tablespoon cocoa powder, unsweetened
- 1 large egg
- 1 tablespoon water
- ½ teaspoon baking soda
- 1/3 cup confectioners' erythritol
- 1 tablespoon peanut butter powder
- ½ tablespoon melted salted butter or coconut oil
- ¾ teaspoon pure vanilla extract
- 2 tablespoons sugar free dark chocolate baking chips

**Method:**

1. Switch on your oven and let it preheat to 35 0° F.
2. Place a 6-count silicone muffin pan on a rimmed baking sheet.
3. Add almond butter, cocoa powder, egg, water, baking soda, erythritol, peanut butter, butter and vanilla extract into a bowl.
4. Beat with an electric hand mixer until well incorporated. You will end up having a thick batter.

5. Add chocolate chips and fold gently.
6. Spoon into the muffin cups.
7. Place baking sheet along with the muffin pan in the oven.
8. Let it bake for 11 minutes.
9. When done, remove the muffin cups and cool completely on a cooling rack.
10. Loosen the edges of the muffin and invert onto a plate.
11. Serve.(**figure. 20**)

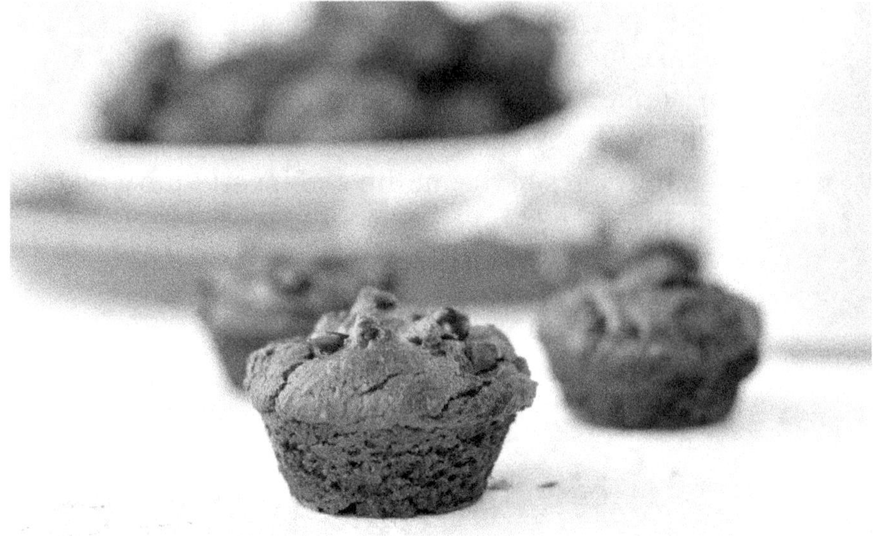

**Figure 20.  Keto Chocolate Muffins.**

## Conclusion

As you reach the end of this book, I would like to thank you for choosing this book. A lot of research has been put into it to give you useful and accurate information.

Once you begin the keto diet, you will understand why it is advocated instead of other diets. It will help you eat well and live better as you keep at it. All the recipes given here are simple and delicious at the same time. You can try them all out and see that your appetite will be sated. There are a lot more keto recipes that you can try out or even create yourself.

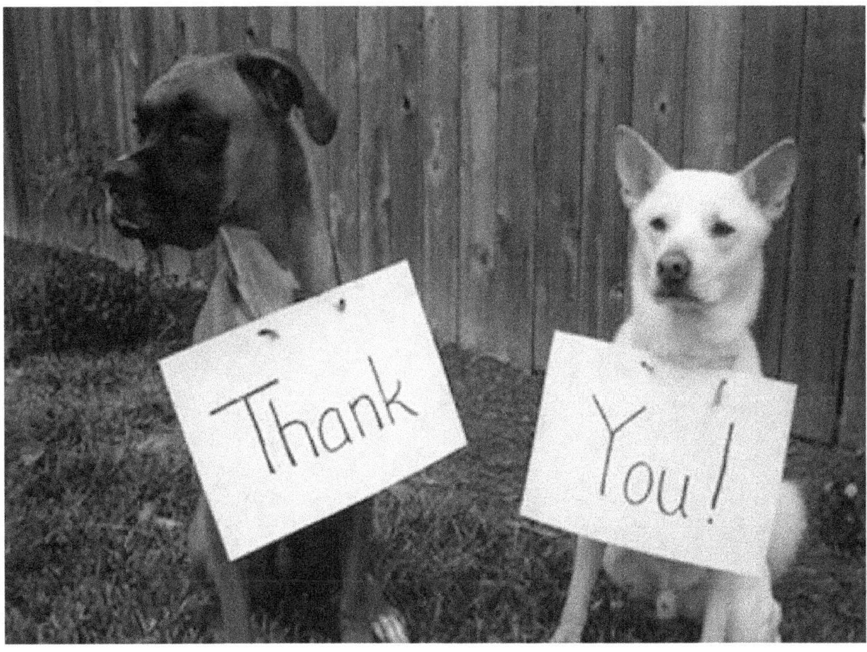


Finally, if you enjoyed this book OR not as the case may be, would you be willing to leave a review? I'd like to ask kindly, PLEASE do leave a review for this book on Amazon. Every, sentence of that review however "good" or "bad" will help us indie authors carve out a career as a creative professional. It'd be greatly appreciated!

GO TO https://amzn.to/2FXbDTc, to leave a review for this book on Amazon!


Thank you and good luck!